# How Not to Gain Weight After Quitting Smoking
## by Andreas Michaelides

How Not to Gain Weight After Quitting Smoking
ISBN: 978-9963-277-12-4
Cyprus Library.
www.cypruslibrary.gov.cy

**Table of Contents**

Find more about me and my
books  at my webpage
http://www.thirsty4health.com

# About the Author

Andreas was born in Athens, the city that gave birth to Democracy, in Greece, the country that taught to the world how to live, think, and have fun. He grew up in the beautiful island of Cyprus.

With both of his parents bibliophiles (and his father a high school teacher), Andreas grew up with a love and appreciation for literature. In addition to the books he borrowed from the school library, a stack of encyclopedias taught him about the world. A history lover from age 13, he devoured the memoirs of Winston Churchill and Charles de Gaul, and by age 17, he had read all of Julius Vern's books.

After serving his country for 26 months immediately after finishing high school, Andreas studied in Patra, Greece to become a computer engineer. With his Master of Computer Engineering and Informatics, he began working in the Informatics Department of the local university hospital, and started reading again with a vengeance.

In 2004, Andreas authored his first book, a historical novel that has not yet seen the light of publication. Leaving it unpublished made him feel like a failure, but a lot has changed since then. Eleven years later, he has successfully quit smoking and has been smoke-free for the past six years. He has also started running again and managed to lose 26 kg (57 lbs).

Andreas has run three marathons, as well as many half-marathons and other shorter races. His love for running is what renewed him and actually saved his life.

Multiple medical problems pushed Andreas to research and experiment with a plant-based diet; since 2013 he is following a whole plant based diet.

In addition to running, Andreas enjoys hiking, cycling, playing basketball, camping, photography, and going out with friends and family and having a good time.

## Prologue.

The few courageous and brave people who told me to quit smoking in the past because it is not good for me are the people who I remember fondly now 7 years after I took my last cigarette and they are probably the ones I really appreciate the most. They were and some still are my best friends.

All the others who said nothing to me while I was poisoning myself and other people around me with secondhand smoking, either because they didn't care if I was a pitiful drug addict or they just didn't care at all about me are forgotten in my oblivious memory.

Some of them saw it as a bad habit so they didn't bother to say anything, and others saw it as my choice to smoke, like I wanted to smoke. Let me tell you something as a former smoker of cigs and now that I see things more clearly. No one wants to smoke; it's a way to administrate a drug in your system, namely nicotine, and it has an iron grip on you!

Anyway, not to get sidetracked here, I really admire those people who were telling me to stop smoking because they are the ones who actually really care about me. Of course, back then, I wanted to rip their throats out because as I saw it, they were interfering with my life.

## Help Smokers Quit…

Thoughts of anger and defensive attitude were in my head and it manifested clearly in my body posture. *Who are you to tell me what to do? I am an adult, I know what I am doing, I like smoking, It's my right to smoke* and other idiotic rationalizations I would present as arguments; not so much to convince other people or the persons telling me to quit but mostly myself so I can keep smoking without having the ethical burden of knowing that I was basically committing a slow paced suicide.

That's why today, whenever I see someone smoking, I tell him or her to stop in their face and I explain the dangers to them. I give the tips on how to stop smoking, I tell them stories from my own experience because I want to help as many people I can. I know that they are boiling inside, some of them are offended, and I tell them that in their face again! I tell them I had the same exactly feelings and attitude towards people who were telling me to stop smoking years ago.

## *Smoking Economics…*

Another reason I want to help people stop smoking, besides their health, which is paramount and number one in my list, is you are saving a lot of money by stopping smoking. It's money that you can spend in more healthy activities instead of funding corporations like Big Tobacco which only researches and invents more poisonous ways to hook young people onto nicotine.

## *Conspiracy Theories?*

Also, what I am about to say might sound stupid but unfortunately, modern societies and societies that democracy, they really don't have any. The countries are run and controlled by the super rich and they have situated rotten politicians in key places to do their dirty work. It doesn't matter if you vote for candidate A, B, or C, which is really rare because it's usually always two candidates. Isn't that a bit convenient, like we would have a problem deciding between 5 or 10 candidates; it has to be two for some reason.
I mean, we have like a zillion different tastes and flavors for candy but as far as our political future is concerned, we usually only have two political parties in most countries.

## *Take the Power…*

Anyway, by stopping smoking, you stop funding big companies and corporations. You deny them money, which is the only item of business they care about; you cut their blood line and dry them out!

It would be nice if they only took your money when they were selling you something and it was beneficial for you, and had a healthy effect on your body and your mental health, but every now and then, a bank will collapse and instead, the governments of this planet make a serious inquiry and punish and put the persons or the institutions responsible for the collapse and the embezzlement of money in jail. Then the governments come to the rescue and bail out the banks! Guess who is paying for that bail out? The taxpayer, you and me, my friends!

## *Food for Thought...*

So, basically, think about this, about 1 billion people on this planet smoke! If all those people stopped smoking, we would take the power from big tobacco and actually change the way this planet operates and functions and it would surely be for the best.

They will have nothing to sell, people will not get sick so the drug companies will lose a lot of money from manufacturing drugs that only manage symptoms of illness that are derived from or are caused from tobacco smoking. Get the picture?

When you stop smoking, you get your health back, you have money out of the blue to use and manage whatever way you fancy and more importantly, you take money away from lobbyists and big corporations that only they care about making themselves richer without giving any consideration to the working man.

## *Government Hypocrisy*

You think the governments increase the price of cigs and add more taxes because they want to help smokers quit? Hell no, they know they are dealing with an addiction. A smoker will pay anything to get their fix.

When I was a smoker, and it happened to be 2 a.m., all hell broke loose if I was out of cigs. I would walk kilometers to find a kiosk open to buy cigs. Nothing stopped me from getting my fix!

Sometimes I would be smoking the last cig of my packet and if the cig somehow fell on the ground, and there were a few more drags on that cig, I would not even think about it. I would pick that cig from the dirty road and continue smoking it like nothing happened. I was a drug addict! Now that I am thinking it, I am shivering to my bones of how much of an out of control junkie I was.

Drug addicts don't care about how expensive their drug is. They are addicted. Reasoning is not the governing force in their life, it's the addiction.

## *Tobacco Taxes...*

Wake up. The governments of this planet know that taxing cigs is money they will get for sure, 100%, every last dime! That's why they don't outlaw smoking. Do you know how easy it is to ban smoking and nicotine use? They did it with other so-called hard drugs, why can't they do it with nicotine? It's not that they can't, they simply won't. I tell you why, and there are two reasons. One, they need a legal drug to put people in addiction. Addicted people are more easily manipulated and controlled. And, two, yes, you guessed it, money!

Governments are run by rotten politicians, politicians who worked for big tobacco at some point or when they retire, they will go back to work for big tobacco.

People smoke, they get sick, then they start giving their hard earned money to Big Pharmaceutical companies, also controlled rotten politicians. Then you have BIG JUNK FOOD industries that do the same thing. They sell people products full of sugar and fat and salt that will make them sick later and they also have rotten politicians and lobbyists working for them to make sure their products (poisons) are even introduced to kids' school cafeterias!

That's why they don't ban nicotine use. I mean, it would stand to reason that it would be smarter to ban and illegalize a drug that kills more people annually than all the so-called illegal drugs put together!

## *Obesity Crisis...*

There is a reason kids around the world are obese and fat by the age of 9! They start them eating junk food from schools. (mention the documentary you saw the other day on Netflix about this matter)
Because BIG-TOBACCO, BIG-PHARMA and BIG-JUNK FOOD control the governments. The people do not hear the truth about what is healthy or not. We are bombarded with misinformation and half-truths so much that people don't know what to follow anymore.

## *The 'Quitting Smoking is Hard' Myth...*

One such misinformation and lies is that quitting smoking is impossible, that only a small percentage of the population can pull it off. Lies, all of it. Of course they want you to believe that quitting smoking is impossible. I used to believe that myself and after a few failed attempts, I almost accepted that I was going to die from smoking because, hey, look, all the health organizations say it's really hard. The reason they want you to believe that is twofold. One, they want you to continue smoking. They don't care, as long you smoke. The tobacco companies are making money and some of that money goes as taxes to the government; it doesn't matter if the tobacco companies make money or the government makes money they are the same coin with two faces. The second reason is to trap you in NRT (Nicotine Replacement Therapies) scenarios. Big –PHARMA, through sheer lobbying, managed to convince the medical sectors of many countries that introducing nicotine to a smoker with an alternative method is a therapy for quitting smoking!
Yes, sure, you quit the act of smoking, taking a cig, putting it in your mouth, lighting it, and then taking a puff. ***You don't do that anymore but you still are a nicotine addict!***

It's the addiction that many smokers wants to get rid of, not the delivery method.

## NRTs, What a Hoax...

There are so many other delivery methods now like vapors, electronic cigs, sprays, candies, gums, pipes; the list is long!
They manage to trick people into that thinking that switching from cigs to NRTs will help them quit smoking.
It's like telling an alcoholic, "Hey, man, we start you on Monday with 10 glasses of whiskey and every day that passes, we will remove a glass until you won't drink any alcohol anymore!"
Any former alcoholic is laughing right now. The way you quit an addiction is to stop putting the substance that creates the addiction into your body. The best, easiest, cheapest, and healthiest way to quit any addiction is going Cold Turkey and I am adamant on this.
My first attempt was with nicotine patches. It ended up in a catastrophic failure, because NRTs like nicotine patches doesn't cure the cause of the condition or the illness, it only manages symptoms, like all drugs made by pharmaceutical companies. I mean, think about it, if the drugs cure the cause of the disease, you wouldn't have to buy their drugs anymore. Where is the profit in that, right?

## Cold Turkey is Gold in My Book...

That's how the majority of ex-smokers stop smoking and that's how I stopped smoking 7 years ago. You simply stop smoking, that's how simple it is!
And for the record, it's not hard to stop smoking and it's not impossible either. There are more ex-smokers right now on this planet than smokers. That's not a measly 7% of people managing to remain smoke-free like they want you to believe, that's 50%. I don't know about you but that's a big number. That means that 1 out 2 people successfully manage to quit smoking and as I said, Cold Turkey is the best method to do that.

Another thing they use to scare smokers away from attempting to stop smoking is by saying that if you stop smoking, you will gain weight, implying that it definitely is going to happen.

Yeah, sure, you gain weight if you are ignorant and don't educate yourself about it, like me 7 years ago.

## *Weight Gain After Quitting…*

I wrote in many of my articles on my blog about not worrying about any weight gain during the quitting process because the stress of the quit is enough for you to worry about. You don't need any more stress or other things to worry about, like what are you going to eat while you are quitting smoking.

I am going to support this advice with two arguments.

First, you don't gain weight because you stop smoking, you gain weight because, in very simple terms, you eat more calories than you burn.

You gain weight because you replaced nicotine with food.

If you need 2,000 calories every day and you eat 2,500 instead, then that's 3,500 excess calories per week and that's about a pound of week extra weight on your body!

## *Dietary Choices and Exercise Habits…*

Second, your dietary and exercise lifestyle will determine if you are going to gain more weight and your dietary choices are far more important than your exercise regime.

If you eat junk food, then you will replace the calories you were getting through smoking with junk food!

If you have a healthier dietary situation going for you, then you replace the extra calorie because of quitting smoking with much healthier, leaner choices and you won't gain so much weight.

It's your mindset that will determine if you are going to gain weight or not.

I am giving my life experience as an example so I make what I mean clearer.

## *Will You Gain Weight or Not?*

I want to repeat this because I think it's a very serious reason many smokers, and I was one of them, never go through the process of quitting smoking and that is that they are afraid that once they quit smoking, they will gain weight, that they will get fat and obese, and they prefer to keep smoking!

It is true that many people gain weight after they quit smoking. Some of them gain little weight, some of them gain a medium share of pounds, and some of them, like me, gain a lot of weight.

The majority of people do not gain a lot of weight. Studies have shown that the average weight gain of is about 5 pounds (2.3kg).That's nothing!

Of the people who quit smoking, about 4% manage to gain weight in the area of 20 pounds and more. Sadly, I belonged to that category.

There are many reasons that drive people to indulge and binge on food after smoking. I was one who fell for the food trap.

One reason is that I used food as a way to continue the mechanical movements I was doing with the cigarettes. I replaced the cigs with food, and I replaced the lighter or the matches with holding a can of soda. Basically, I replaced nicotine with food.

## *Ahhh, Dopamine…*

Every time I would smoke a cig, the nicotine would initiate a process where dopamine would give me pleasurable sensations. I replaced those nicotine generated dopamine sensations with food generated dopamine sensations. It was not the same but it was better than nothing.

I had this mentality that because I managed to quit smoking, I could pat myself on the back by rewarding myself and my reward was I could eat whatever I wanted because I deserved it!

It would be a perfect scenario if I had the metabolism of Captain America but unfortunately, my metabolism started to become slower even when I was a smoker. The myth that when you stop smoking, it makes your metabolism slower is a red herring.

Studies have shown that Basal Metabolic Rate (BMR) isn't really affected that much when we stop smoking.

## *Subconscious Knowledge…*

Now I always knew that smoking was not good for me and in the back of my mind, I always thought it was a bad habit that I could easily stop whenever I desired.

I knew about nicotine but it just didn't register or click in my head to make the connection that the reason I was smoking was because I was a nicotine addict. And that I was no different than an alcoholic, cocaine user, or heroin user. The only difference, except for the alcohol, is it was not illegal to use my drug! That's the only difference.

So, yes, I saw a couple of friends of mine in Greece and also a few other acquaintances who had successfully quit smoking and all of them gained a lot of weight. So, yes, I am admitting that back then, one of the reasons I didn't try to stop smoking was the fear of gaining weight.

The fear of heart attack, stroke, both of which can bring sudden death by the way, the fear of lung, mouth, esophageal cancer, pulmonary obstructions, or emphysema did not scare me at all because I was basically a stupid little ignorant man.

I would smoke with vengeance, putting myself in danger every time I was taking a puff. Literally every time a smoker takes a puff, it might be the last thing he will ever do! Take a puff, then poof, he or she is dead!

## *Failed Attempts…*

I had many failed attempts, which I mentioned in my first book, *Thirsty for Health*, in one of my latest books, 16 Common Smoking Rationalizations, Recognized, Analyzed and Ultimate Destroyed! ,and in a lot of my smoking articles on my blog.

Of course, the only attempt that really counts for me is the one I did 7 years ago and it is still my successful quit because I haven't smoke since!

I don't know if I was born with it, picked it from my family environment, or learned it in school, or a variation of all them, but I have a good ability or innate characteristic in that I tend to learn from my mistakes and failures and I strive to be better and more successful the next time I attempt to do something similar.

## *Learning Through Failure….*

So all of my previous attempts to quit smoking were not in vain. I learned that smoking is not just a bad habit, that something more sinister was there under the surface of my hypnotized mind and I needed to search more.

With every failed attempt, my resolve was getting stronger. Of course, I was disappointed with every failed quit but I was learning and making sure I wouldn't make the same mistakes on my next attempt.

Unfortunately, there are people who attempt to quit and fail and then don't try again, either because they are weak or refuse to get into the process of actually learning from their failures and mistakes.

That's the beauty of the human mind and spirit, we learn through our mistakes and we better ourselves dramatically using this situation.

## *Unhealthy Situations…*

As I said earlier, when I was 31 years old, I was about 154 pounds (70 kg) and I was a chain smoker, I had zero exercise, and I was eating heavily processed food (salt, sugar, fat) namely fast food, junk food, and my metabolism managed to preserve that weight until I was 34.When I reached that age and continued the same dietary and lack of exercise lifestyle, I gained another 22 pounds in one year. The reason I gained 22 pounds in one year was because it was the year I left Greece and came back to

Cyprus. I was stressed because I didn't have a steady job, I was working from 5 a.m. until midnight, I was doing 3 to 4 jobs at the same time, and I was always eating junk food. And guess what? I was smoking at the same time as well, so this stupid myth that smoking helps you lose weight or helps you not to gain weight is idiotic and doesn't apply.

Let me repeat it, you gain weight if you eat more calories than you can burn and it gets worse if your dietary preferences are shitty as well (junk food, processed food, etc.).

## *How Smoking Makes You Gain Weight...*

Now here is a good time to tell you how smoking actually is responsible for gaining weight, not losing weight, and that's what happened with me.

The feelings of hunger and nicotine withdrawal symptoms are similar and in time, as your body becomes more immune to the effect of nicotine, you have this constant feeling of hunger that you don't know how to satisfy because you don't know if you are hungry or in need of nicotine. I was like that. I would have this feeling and I didn't know what to do, so I end up smoking as much as my pocket could afford and my lungs could take, and when I was not smoking, I would be eating.

That's why smoking and eating is associated with each other so much. I mean, you will see that after they eat, smokers usually light up a cig.

When you eat and you really need to smoke or when you smoke and you really need to eat are so messed up in a smoker's life, he ends up gaining weight because he doesn't know when to satisfy the two. That's what happened with me at some point, ending up gaining 22 pounds while smoking!

## *Helpful Conclusions...*

This experience helped me understand and see that smoking doesn't help you reduce weight or keep you thin. I saw firsthand that it was a myth and a hoax.

Having that in mind, it was easier for me to go ahead this time and stop smoking where as in the past, I didn't even attempt to quit smoking because of fear of gaining weight. Now that fear was not a reality for me anymore.

Another reason I gained weight while I was smoking was the fact that smoking poisons your body, especially your lungs, restricting you from any athletic activities like running or walking, for example. Both are a very effective way of burning calories. For every mile ran, an average man burns about 100 calories!

Cycling, swimming, or playing football, basketball, ping pong, or tennis are all activities that help a person to boost their metabolism. It also strengthens our immune systems and makes them healthier and also helps us burn calories.

Smokers do not do that because their lungs are a mess and they are slowly rendered useless and destroyed by the 4,000 chemicals that are in the cigarette.

So there you go, junk food, full of empty calories, eating more calories than you burn, and no exercise to burn any more calories is why you gain weight, not because you stop smoking or you smoke.

It doesn't matter if you are a smoker or non-smoker, weight gain at its core is more calories in than calories out.

## Nicotine Feeding...

Now let me tell you a few things about how smoking, and namely nicotine, messes us up as far as weight loss is concerned.

When you take a puff, nicotine, in very simple terms, is bullying our liver into releasing glucose and fat into your blood stream, which it has stored inside it. This intravenous feeding is what tricks our brain. Nicotine, with this ability to command the liver to elevate the body's blood sugar levels, is what makes our brain think that we have already eaten so we don't feel the signs of hunger.

Hunger starts to kick in when our glucose blood levels are down and when our stomach is empty. In very simple words, the process goes like this.

14

We eat until we fill our stomach, then the stomach sends a signal to our brain to tell it that we are full. But that signal takes 20minutes to reach the brain, which is why it's important to chew our food slow and eat at a pleasant pace so our feeding time will correspond with the 20 minute delay.

For example, if you gulp your food in 5 minutes, you filled your stomach, but the message that will inform the brain that we are full and satisfied will reach the brain 15 minutes later.

So, basically, we keep eating because the message of satisfaction hasn't reach the brain yet to tell us stop eating!

After we eat something, it takes about 20 to 30 minutes for the nutrients and the glucose to enter our bloodstream.

With nicotine, we achieve the same effect but not in 20 minutes. It is much, much faster, we are talking about seconds!

## *Messy Feeding Method…*

So imagine a smoker doing this thing to themselves for years. Every time they were hungry, instead of eating like a normal person does, they would smoke a cig and the hunger would go away because nicotine tricked their brain into thinking that they had already eaten.

Smoking doesn't help you maintain your weight or lose weight, it kills you from the inside out and destroys the feeding mechanisms of your body, with all the side effects that entails.

When you feel hunger in your stomach, you should feed yourself properly, not deplete your liver's glucose storage! That's the most unnatural thing to do! It is called glucose storage for a reason, it is there to feed the brain and our nervous system, not to be released on command so you will stop feeling hungry!

Using nicotine as a hunger cessation mechanism puts you in danger of heart attack, stroke, lung cancer, limp amputation, and so many other "wonderful benefits" smoking offers to you!

Of course, there are only a number of cigs you can smoke and get away with it. At some point, the brain realizes that you need to eat real food! So you have to eat! And when you eat, you might eat more calories than you burn and that's how you gain weight, not because you are going to stop smoking.

## *A Year After Quitting…*

In April 2010, I took a really hard look at myself after getting out of the shower and I did not like what I saw. I was 44 pounds overweight! I put on 20 of those pounds while I was a smoker and the rest after I quit smoking!

I decided to quit smoking for many reasons. I always knew it was bad for me but for a number of reasons, not ready, being ignorant that I was a drug addict, how the addiction works, etc., I couldn't find the way that would allow me to commit and take the decision to remove the addiction from my life.

What made me make the decision and make the commitment was the fact that I really got sick and tired of smoking. I was disgusted by myself and it drove me to take action. I realized that if I continued down this path, I would be dead or crippled for life. My life as I knew it, or as I wished it to be, was not going to be a reality and that scared me the most.

Same approach and same philosophy happened with me being overweight and flirting with obesity. I didn't like what I saw in the mirror and I got sick and tired of looking like that so I decided to take action like I did with smoking.

Funny thing is that when I decided to stop smoking, in the back of my mind, and to be honest until recently, it was this notion and to some extent a belief, that is was really hard to stop smoking and I was really lucky that I managed to quit, that I belonged to that 7% of the population that manages to quit smoking.

As I explained earlier, this is not the truth. It's easy to stop smoking, the hard part is to remain smoke-free!

On the contrary, me eating like a pig and doing no exercise at all was not something that registered as something unhealthy.

Well, it is better to be slightly overweight than being slim and smoke like a chimney! I mean, I would have had to put an extra 75 pounds to reach the same risk level of a smoker who smokes a pack a day. In other words, to reach the same overload condition nicotine puts on my heart, I would have had to gain another 75 pounds.

Well, having said that, being overweight is not a healthy way of living either. The irony about my extra pounds was that back then, I thought that shedding the pounds would be easy as pie. The statistics were against me though, and of course, I didn't know that.

It turns out that only 4% of the people who lose the extra pounds manage to keep them off! That's 4%, now compare that with 50% of successful chances of quitting smoking and you get an idea of the reality I was not aware a few years ago.

That's how people get exploited and scammed. A task of quitting smoking, when applied correctly (using Cold Turkey Method), is so easy, but is presented by the media(controlled by BIG-industries) as impossible to do. Quitting smoking is hard, they say. To quit smoking is really hard to achieve, so hard that you must use prescription drugs or NRTs (Nicotine Replacement Therapies).

On the other hand, the task of losing weight and keeping the pounds off, which is really hard to do, is presented like something really easy and something you can do in a few days, like those pounds didn't take years to accumulate! If they really showed people the proper way to keep the weight off, then they wouldn't be selling all the diets that don't work, selling all the gymnastic equipment that do not really help any, taking people's money and plunging them into depression even more.

## _A Vicious Cycle..._

Because people think that smoking helps them lose weight, some ex-smokers, after trying a number of yo-yo diets or gadgets that didn't do anything to their waistline, they start smoking again, thinking it will help them lose weight. That's maybe the biggest mistake an overweight ex-smoker can make.

The pounds will not go away because smoking doesn't help you lose weight. As I explained earlier, it makes you gain weight and now you are in double danger for heart attack, stroke, and other diseases like lung cancer, colorectal cancer, Type 2 diabetes, etc.!

If you are an ex-smoker, and you are overweight and you want to lose weight, then you need first to change your way of thinking and then adopt a lifestyle, not a diet, which will help you lose weight safely, gradually, and permanently.

The way I did it, as I describe it in my book, *How I Lost 44 Pounds and Never Gained Them Back Using a Plant-based Diet* is as the title says. I adopted a plant-based diet and I stick with it and it works.

Besides the nutritional aspect of the whole endeavor, I started running again and one of the reasons I wrote my book, *How to Train and Finish Your First 5k Race*, is to show and help people see that it is not hard or impossible to adopt athletics into your life and to also show you the benefits of them.

That's how I lost 44 pounds and never gained them back. I changed my mindset, I adopted a healthier nutritional lifestyle, and I started exercising.

## *Addictions....*

I need to mention three names here because I really want to honor these three men. They helped immensely, not so much to quit smoking but after I quit smoking, to understand the depth of my addiction, which help me prisoner for 16years, the most productive years of my life from the age of 19 until the age of 35!

These three guys help me recognize all the feelings, psychological urges, physiological urges, social triggers, bad smoking dreams, and so many other aspects of being a smoker and also being an ex-smoker. They really helped put my smoking journey in perspective from the moment I took that first puff 23 years ago until the moment I took the last puff from the tube of death 7 years ago.

## *My Three "Smoking" Musketeers*

*Allen Carr.*† – Died from Lung Cancer on November 29, 2006, at age 72. God rest his soul.

https://www.allencarr.com/
YouTube videos– There are 199 of them!
https://www.amazon.com/Allen-
Carr/e/B001XSUEK4/ref=sr_tc_2_0?qid=1472469181&sr=1-2-
ent

### *John R. Polito*
Nicotine Cessation Educator and Director & Founder
WhyQuit.com
http://whyquit.com/JohnBio.html
YouTube channel
Book, *Freedom from Nicotine – A Journey Home* – completely
free to download.
Amazon page of the book (https://www.amazon.com/Freedom-
Nicotine-John-R-Polito-
ebook/dp/B008UAPXWC/ref=sr_1_1?ie=UTF8&qid=14786332
94&sr=8-1&keywords=John+R.+Polito)   You can buy it and
give it as a gift to a smoker you know.

### *Joel Spitzer*

Director of Education
http://whyquit.com/joel/whyquitbio.htm
Book, *Never Take Another Puff* – completely free to download.
YouTube channel
Quit Smoking Library

## *In the Process of Quitting…*

If you are thinking of quitting smoking, then I have the
following advice to you. I wish someone told me this
information when I did my successful quit 7years ago; I am sure
my quit would have been easier and I also wouldn't end up being
22 pounds heavier.
It's up to you to use this information for your benefit. You are
lucky that I got fat after quitting smoking because if I didn't, I
would have probably never learned what it takes to lose weight
effectively, safely, and permanently, and I wouldn't be here

sharing it with you with the hope that I would make a difference in your lives and in the life of this planet.

## *First 72 Hours...*

The first 72 hours are crucial for your quit. The important thing to remember is not to alter anything from your daily routine. Do not go and close yourself in your apartment or your house and keep yourself away from any social gatherings or contacts.

You need to quit smoking while doing the things you did but now you need to train yourself that you will do them from now on without smoking.

Now, the first three days, you may have nicotine withdrawal symptoms. Notice that I said may' you might have them but you might not have them at all. How many cigs you smoked or how many years you smoked are irrelevant with the severity of your withdrawal symptoms.

Being a heavy smoker or a light smoker, or smoking for 3 months or 30 years does not have analogous withdrawal symptoms; it plays a bigger role in social triggers after you shed the nicotine out of your body.

Someone who is a smoker for 30 years has much more ingrained social associations with smoking and living compared to someone who only smoked for 6 months, but as for the physiological effects of nicotine withdrawal, you might have them for the first three days, and you might not. You might have severe or mild but most people are in between, they have a medium level and intensity of withdrawal symptoms.

## *My First 72 Hours...*

My first 72 hours were a medium-intensity and I had mild severity symptoms. Of course, back then, I had no idea about the fact that the first 72 hours are critical because the bulk of the nicotine is leaving your body and leaves your body completely in two weeks!

I, on the other hand, read back then that nicotine needs 3 weeks to leave the body and I set a goal in my mind that if I manage to not smoke for 3 weeks, then I would be free of smoking and I would not have any reason to smoke anymore.

It worked for me but think how easy it would be for me if I had this information available back then. The information, of course, was there, I just didn't search or research to find them.

Now as I have already mentioned, because nicotine is a hunger depressant, when you stop smoking and nicotine is leaving your body, and you are not eating adequately, you might feel a drop in your glucose blood levels, which will lead to headaches and other effects like shaking or irritability. Therefore, in the first three days, it is a good tactic to drink lots of natural, fresh squeezed juices, which will help you maintain your blood sugar in normal levels.

Also, by drinking lots of juices for the first three days, you are not going to feel hungry all the time and you will not eat all the time!

Also, you are setting an example for your body, you are giving it time to recuperate from the unnatural way it was getting glucose all these years, and training your body to get glucose from food rather than from the stimulation of you liver through nicotine.

Do you know what I did the first three days of my quit? I drank lots of sodas and ice teas full of sugar. I ate lots of chocolates, croissants, potato chips, and lots and lots of Pringles. I remember that I was devouring them, and on top of that, I was eating three large meals a day, breakfast, lunch, and dinner!

So it is important to drink lots of juices, especially cranberry juice, for the first three days. Cranberry juice and other fresh juices without any added sugars or preservatives make our urine more acidic.

Our body takes nicotine from our blood stream and sends it to our urine to make it more alkaline, resulting in the elimination of nicotine of our body at a faster pace.

So drinking fresh squeezed juices helps us in two ways. It helps to prevent sugar cravings and removes nicotine from our body faster.

## *What I Learned by Adopting a Plant-based Diet...*

What I am going to tell you is paramount and the most important information I have for you as weight control after you quit smoking. If you are like me, then you probably replaced and substituted nicotine with food.

It is a "natural" thing to do because after the third day of your quit, your sense of smell starts to work again and your taste buds are functioning better, so, naturally, food smells and tastes better. I bet your coffee will taste more aromatic and full now!

So it's only natural to indulge in binge eating. Don't do that, do not do what I did and end up being dangerously flirting with obesity. It took me 4 years to gradually lose that weight.

It took me 3 weeks to get rid of smoking but took me 4 years to lose the weight safely and naturally and never gain them back.

So what you need to do is do two basic and very important things.

First, you need to sit and calculate how many calories you were eating(a rough estimate) when you were a smoker and then break those calories to 5 or 6 small meals a day. This way, you will have your glucose blood levels satisfied all the time and you want be feeling hungry or tempted to binge.

Second, you need to replace empty calories with dense caloric food that are mostly plant-based.

A few examples so you understand what I am talking about. If you eat 200 calories worth of chicken, you will only put about 115 grams in your stomach, and you will need a lot more chicken to fill it up because if you don't, you will still be hungry because you need to fill your stomach at least 50% for the brain to send the signal so you stop eating.

So instead of eating animal-based products like meat, dairy products, fish, and seafood, and processed food, which has lots of calories but small volume, replace them with plant-based ones that have fewer calories per volume.

But if you eat 200 calories worth of boiled potatoes, you will put 229 grams of food in your stomach! Get the picture? By replacing animal products with plant-based products, you can eat more (quantity) but with less calories, resulting in an effective way to control your weight.

Also, prefer boiled over fried. Oils, whether animal- or plant-based, are mostly fat and you should stay away from them.

Eat lots of vegetables and fruits. They are bulky with fiber, keep you full for longer, and you don't have to binge with sweets or candies or other kinds of junk food.

Put boiled beans, boiled potatoes, and boiled beets in your salads. Prefer vinegar instead of olive oils.

Eat a lot of legumes. They are full of nutrients and they release the glucose into your blood slowly and for longer periods of time.

Stay away from white sugar, white rice, white salt (water retention and high blood pressure), and white flour.

Limit processed and refined food. They offer empty calories and you need to eat a lot of them.

Be extra careful with sugar. Replace it with stevia (a zero caloric sweetener). You can use agave nectar instead of honey; it doesn't spike your blood sugar level like honey does, and it tastes like honey!

Use blackstrap molasses and dates as sweeteners, too; they are highly nutritious also.

Drink lots of water, instead of sodas or other processed beverages.

## *Psychological Triggers...*

While I was having my coffee, I would smoke. After sex, I would usually smoke. When I was having an alcoholic drink, I would smoke and, of course, after I finished a meal, the first thing I would do without even thinking was to get up from the table and reach for my pack of cigs. I would take one, put it in my mouth, light it using my favorite Zippo lighter, and smoke happily, lost in my ignorant bliss of death and destruction of my body and soul.

After I stopped smoking, the thing I did not manage to do, and it was one of the reasons I gained so much weight was that I replaced smoking after food with sweet desserts!

After I finished eating, instead of smoking, I would eat an ice cream or two, or a few slices of the super tasty apple pie made by my mother. I didn't eat fruits, which would be a healthier alternative! Processed or refined food were adding extra unburned calories on my waistline, accumulating slowly week after week.

You would think it is hard to deconstruct how I gain those 22 pounds in a year but if you analyze it, it comes to very few unburned calories a day to reach the magic 22.

A pound has 3,500 calories. Multiply that by 22, and we have 77,000 calories. Divide that by 52, which are the weeks in a year, and we have 1,480 calories. Divide that by 7, which is the days of a week, and we have about 211 calories a day!

So I was eating 211 calories a day more than I was burning! 211 calories is a slice of apple pie or an ice cream, or… or… or…you get the picture?

## *What You Can Do…*

You need to train yourself to acquire and apply healthy ending meal cues. For example, after you finish eating, get up and go for a walk. If you can't get up from the table, make sure you don't have any desserts or sweets or any other kind of food near you. Use a toothpick to clean your teeth, meditate by taking long breaths and slow exhalations, brush your teeth, or chew a non-sugar gum. These are some of the things you can do after eating to replace the smoking trigger and avoid eating calories.

## *Start Exercising…*

Start exercising the soonest you can! Go see your doctor and tell him/her that you want to start walking, and that you wish to turn to running in the future.

Your doctor will probably give you physical and cardiograph to check out the condition of your heart. Once you get the green light, wear your walking shoes and go out there and start moving as I describe in my book, *How to Train and Finish Your First 5k Race*. Start by walking at a regular pace, and walk until you stay out of breath. Time yourself from the moment you started walking until the time you were out of breath and note that time as your current base. For example, if it took you 10 minutes from start to shortness of breath, then that's your endurance current ability. I know, sad but true, but it's in your hands, actually, in your legs, to make that time and distance better and longer.

Start walking every other day for 10 minutes for 3 weeks. When the fourth week comes, you will notice that you can walk more than 10 minutes without shortness of breath. Excellent! Congratulations, you just became fitter and you made your metabolism faster for sure.

Continue increasing your walking time. Listen to your body, it will tell you when it's ready to go further or faster or both.

At some point, you will want to start running and that's wonderful. Running is one of the best calorie burning exercises you can use to maintain your weight or lose weight.

## *How to Lose Weight...*

You stopped smoking for a while now and you gain a few pounds. Nothing to worry about, or you gain a lot of pounds and you are worrying about it like I was.

Don't worry! What you need to do first is acquire a way of thinking that will enable you to change. You need to change your way of thinking and perception first. If you are going to be successful in losing pounds, you need to change your mind first to sculpt your body the way you want.

You need to open your mind to other possibilities and options, alternatives ways, and paths.

The first thing you need to understand is that you will lose the pounds the way you gain them as far as time is concerned. You didn't gain 20 pounds in three weeks, so why do you believe all these scammers who claim you can lose them in that short

25

amount of time? You didn't gain 5 pounds in a day, it probably took you a month and so on.

So first thing you need to grasp is that to lose weight safely and permanently, you need to lose it gradually and slowly.

If you eat 100 calories less every day, or if you burn 100 calories every day and create a deficit, then in a year, it's 36,500 calories! That's about 10 pounds! Just by creating a deficit of 100 calories every day. Now, that's not hard, is it?

You need to practice with foods. You need to learn a little bit of how many calories the food you eat contains.

I personally use chronometer.com to track my calorie intake. It doesn't give me an exact calorie count but it gives me an estimation and that's how you should go about it. Don't be slaves to calorie counting.

That's one thing, the other is that you have an exercise regime that will enable you to burn that 100 calories easier and also by adopting a plant-based diet as much as you can. I am not asking you to stop animal products but try to increase your plant consumption because as I already mentioned, you will be getting more quantity with less calories.

The cool thing about adopting a plant-based diet and applying an exercise regime at the same time is that I can eat as much as I want without worrying I will gain weight.

## *In a Nutshell...*

Smoking does not help you lose weight, smoking is not the culprit when you gain weight after quitting smoking, and it should not hold you back from attempting to quit smoking. If you are a non-smoker, or an ex-smoker, and you are overweight, for the love of all that is holy, do not start smoking, thinking it will help you lose weight. It won't, you will only put yourself in a double risk of heart attack, strokes, a series of cancers, Type 2 diabetes, limb amputation, and so on!

Drink lots of fresh natural juices made by you with no added sugars or preservatives for the first 3 days of your quit; it will help you with normalizing your blood sugar levels.

Count how many calories you were eating as a smoker and divide those calories into 5 or 6 small meals throughout the day. This way, you will not be hungry all the time and you won't binge on junk food.

Apply an exercise program. It will help you burn calories and maintain your weight. You can consult a trainer and a dietician to help you even more with that.

Replace smoking after food with exercise, a toothpick, brushing your teeth, and so on.

Bottom line, and I leave you with this, make the commitment to educate yourself satisfactorily as to help you lose the pounds you don't want in a healthy and permanent way.

I hope I helped. Have a healthy and happy day!

My warmest regards,

Andreas Michaelides

# *Other books by Andreas Michaelides*

## My weight loss journey: How I lost 44 pounds and never gained them back using a plant based diet

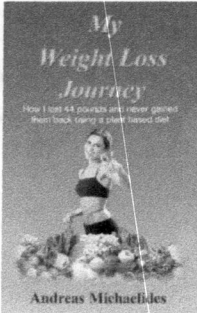

Although I never expected to drag myself out of the house and go for a run, after I finished those first three rounds at the high school track in my village, everything changed. I was so exhausted—which was an indicator of how lacking my physical fitness was—but after all the discomfort, itching, and rash in various places due to friction from excess fat, for the first time, I felt renewed, and memories of running and coming in first place in high school reminded me of how I used to be compared to how I was after those three laps around the track.

It made my eyes water; I was alone in the middle of the track under an April sky full of stars when tears of mixed feelings started pouring down from my eyes. Emotionally and psychologically, it was a turning point for me, and it also made me even more determined to become that lean, mean running machine I used to be. It was right there in that single moment that I saw the path I had to follow.

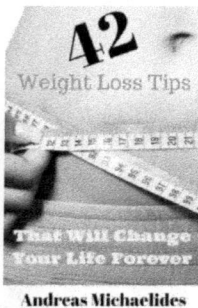

## 42 Weight Loss Tips That Will Change Your Life Forever.

One of the first things I did when I was overweight and decided I had enough was to order from Amazon a lot of books about weight loss, many of them were hocus pocus, others were ok, and some of them were amazing.

That's why in my books, I try to deliver information that the reader, that's you, will find useful and also be able to apply it immediately or at a reasonable pace.

I am a very practical man; I will read the theory as long as I can see the usefulness of it and also the practical applications that it offers.

## *Please write a review.*

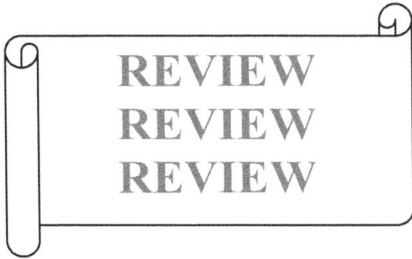

REVIEW
REVIEW
REVIEW

I consider myself as a person that wants to think that I am constantly improving my books, my work and myself. I am always trying to deliver to my readers the best quality and current information out there as my area of interest and expertise is concern which is Health, Nutrition and Exercise.

In order to accomplish that I need feedback from you and the only feedback I know that will help me achieve a relative perfection in all areas of my life is your valuable reviews so I know where I am wrong or where I have made mistakes and errors.

There is no such thing as a perfect book out there, perfection for one person is a sloppy work for other, so in order to satisfy as much as people out there my books need to be updated regularly and it doesn't matter if it is in electronic form (kindle) or paperback form.

If you found this book useful, please leave your review with all your thoughts, don't hold back, it will only take a few minutes of your time.

If you didn't like this book, please let me know by contacting me and I will give my best shot to fix the issue.

Thank you very much,

My warmest regards

Andreas Michaelides

www.ingramcontent.com/pod-product-compliance
Lightning Source LLC
Chambersburg PA
CBHW071036280326
41935CB00011B/1546